Bruno Araújo da Silva Dantas
Jéssica M. A. de Miranda
Gilson de V. Torres

Ageing and quality of life in the community

Bruno Araújo da Silva Dantas
Jéssica M. A. de Miranda
Gilson de V. Torres

Ageing and quality of life in the community

The elderly and the most important aspects of their health

ScienciaScripts

Imprint

Cover image: www.ingimage.com

This book is a translation from the original published under ISBN 978-3-330-76204-6.

Publisher:
Sciencia Scripts
is a trademark of
Dodo Books Indian Ocean Ltd. and OmniScriptum S.R.L publishing group

120 High Road, East Finchley, London, N2 9ED, United Kingdom
Str. Armeneasca 28/1, office 1, Chisinau MD-2012, Republic of Moldova, Europe
Managing Directors: Ieva Konstantinova, Victoria Ursu
info@omniscriptum.com

Printed at: see last page
ISBN: 978-620-8-38303-9

CONTENTS

ACKNOWLEDGEMENTS

We would like to thank all those who collaborated in the development of this research, especially Prof Dr Gilson de Vasconcelos Torres, who provided the knowledge and the right paths for the research.

To the members of the Nursing Procedures Incubator Research Group, who contributed by working as a team, with seriousness and commitment. Within the group, special thanks go to the people who make up the elderly project, who worked hard, with commitment and responsibility, favouring in an important way the process of planning and carrying out activities, as well as the initial data collection of our research.

To Thazia Costa and Thaiza Nobre, who made it possible to contact and get to know the elderly people in the intervention groups, and who were fundamental to the development of the work.

To the elderly people of the Francisco André Group in Igapó, who always welcomed us with affection and satisfaction during the activities carried out in the activity centres.

To the elderly people of the ESF in the Dner neighbourhood and the FACISA Physiotherapy School Clinic, both in Santa Cruz, who always welcomed our team with enthusiasm and satisfaction when we carried out the activities.

CHAPTER 1

Linking ageing and its Quality of Life to the community context

Discussions on health policies for the elderly have been conducted and based on the demographic transition, through global population ageing[1] . In old age, the elderly associate their individual ageing process with the degree of comorbidities and dependency that occur during this process. Thus, the parameters related to this are made up of factors such as body image, autonomy, functionality, family support, mental health and cognition .[2]

Functional decline stands out among the changes that occur in old age, identifying a variable degree of movement limitations, loss of muscle mass, as well as changes in cognitive level, hearing and vision[3] . Lawton and Brody (1969)[4] define functionality by the degree of dependence in carrying out daily activities, attributing functional decline to the inability or difficulty in carrying out these activities.

All of these changes, when associated with the lifestyle habits of the elderly, are predictors of their vulnerability to health risks and their Quality of Life (QoL) .[5]

The World Health Organisation (WHO) defines QoL as the individual perception of human beings with regard to their life situation in a given reality, taking into account a range of values that relate to their goals and expectations[6] . Furthermore, the WHO

also proposes the concept of active ageing, which consists of maintaining the individual's physical, mental and social potential as a strategy for improving QoL in ageing .[7]

Considering the subjectivity of the concept of QoL and the idea of active ageing, the study by Cruz, et al (2013)[8] , shows various proposals for measuring these aspects, based on the main domains that make up QoL. *The Medical Outcomes Study 36-Item Short Form Health Survey* (SF-36) QoL assessment tool has been validated in Brazil and is widely used in various studies, assessing domains such as pain, functional capacity, physical limitations, emotional and social aspects, among others .[8-9]

Turning to the complexity of the concept of QoL, we see that it is directly related to important aspects such as emotional, cognitive, psychological and functional[10] . When faced with such a large number of demands, a multi-professional team is required to ensure comprehensive care for the elderly .[11]

In Brazil, the Family Health Strategy (ESF) is the main way of conducting primary care, characterised by being the first level of complexity of the Unified Health System (SUS), i.e. the Brazilian hierarchical health care system. The ESF is represented by a multi-professional team inserted into the socio-cultural scenario of the individual and their family[12] . Within its remit, the policies aimed at the elderly population provide for the various needs of this public, with the aim of promoting health and healthy ageing .[13]

The ESF teams set out to identify the demands inherent in ageing by getting closer to the elderly, through actions such as consultations, home visits and other health promotion and prevention activities[14] . In the midst of the prospects for comprehensive care, the ESF team must remain inserted in the community, seeking to form bonds with the individual and their family, aiming for a relationship of trust for greater effectiveness of the planned actions .[15]

In order to carry out a study with a high level of evidence, it is important to emphasise that the work presented in this book is an initial cross-sectional study of a case-control study, which is part of a large research project entitled "Health Care for the Elderly in the Family Health Strategy in Brazil and Portugal: a proposal for multidimensional evaluation and intervention". International coverage will also be achieved at a later date.

References

1. World Health Organisation (WHO). World Report on Ageing and Health, WHO Library Cataloguing-in-Publication. World Hearth Organisation; 2015.

2. Hein MA, Aragaki SS. Health and ageing: a study of Brazilian master's dissertations (2000-2009). Ciência & Saúde Coletiva. 2012; 17(8): 2141-50.

3. Garatachea N, Galeano HP, Gomar FS, Lozano AS, Luces CF, Morán M, et al. Exercise Attenuates the Major Hallmarks of Aging. Rejuvenation Research. 2015; 18(1): 57-89.

4. Lawton MP, Brody EM. Assessment of Older People: Self-Maintaining and Instrumental Activities of Daily Living. Gerontology. 1969; 9: 179-86.

5. Varela FRA, Ciconelli RM, Campolina AG, Soarez PC. Quality of life evaluation of frail elderly in Campinas, São Paulo. Journal of the Brazilian Medical Association. 2015; 61(5): 423-30.

6. World Health Organisation. The Whoqol Group . The World Health Organisation quality of life assessment (WHOQOL): position paper from the World Health Organisation. Social Science and Medicine, 1995, 10:1403-9.

7. World Health Organisation (WHO). Active aging: a policy framework. World Hearth Organisation; 2002.

8. Cruz LN, Fleck MPA, Oliveira MR, Camey SA, Hoffman JF, Bagattini AM, et al. Health-related quality of life in Brazil: normative data for the SF-36 in a general population sample in the south of the country. Ciência & Saúde Coletiva. 2013; 18(7): 1911-21.

9. Campos MO, Rodrigues Neto JF, Silveira MF, Neves DMR, Vilhena JM, Oliveira JF, et al. Impact of risk factors for chronic non-communicable diseases on quality of life. Ciência & Saúde Coletiva. 2013; 18(3): 873-82.

10. Palgi Y, Shrira A, Zaslavsky O. Quality of life attenuates age-related decline in functional status of older adults. Quality Life Research. 2015; 24: 1835-43.

11. Ferreira FPC, Bansi LO, Paschoal SMP. Elderly care services and home and institutional care strategies. Revista Brasileira de Geriatria Gerontologia. 2014; 17(4): 911-26.

12. Silva LMS. Fernandes MC, Mendes EP, Evangelista NC, Torres RAM. Interdisciplinary work in the Family Health Strategy: focus on care and

management actions. Revista enfermermagem UERJ. 2012; 20(2): 784-8.

13. Brazil. Ministry of Health. Ageing and health of the elderly. Health Care Secretariat. Department of Primary Care. Brasília: Ministry of Health; 2007.

14. Pilger C. Dias JF, Kanawava C, Baratieri T, Carreira L. Understanding of ageing and actions developed by nurses in primary health care. Ciência y Enfermeria. 2013; 19 (1): 61-73.

15. Polaro SHI, Gonçalvez LHT, Alvarez AM. Constructing gerontological practice by nurses from Family Health Strategy Units. Revista Escola de Enfermagem da USP. 2013; 47(1): 160-67.

CHAPTER 2

The complexity of Quality of Life and its aspects

It is clear that the QoL of the elderly is directly influenced by changes and limitations in their routine. These problems generate major concerns on the part of health teams in relation to fitness for daily activities, physical exercise and social interaction, for example .[1-2]

Similarly to the WHO, several other authors define QoL from different perspectives, in which personal, cultural and religious aspects are implicit, as potential influencers of its perception, as well as its impact on the individual's behaviour. In this context, the maintenance of health with its physical, psychological, social and spiritual aspects inherent to human life stands out .[3-4]

In addition to the context of QoL, the presence and increase of risk situations, chronic diseases and other problems during the ageing process is notable. In this sense, vulnerability is an equally important factor in assessing the risk of the elderly, especially .[5]

Accepting the idea that the concept of health is complex and multidimensional, the involvement of the health team becomes essential in the health-disease process of the elderly. In view of the particularities of these individuals, adequate planning is required when intervening in their demands. To this end, the ESF has the elderly population as one of its main targets, with the aim of reorganising care and directing the best quality of service to this public. This system, in turn, gains

supported by operational guidelines and contemplates the doctrinal principles of the SUS .[6]

In Brazil, in accordance with the principles of the SUS, there are public policies aimed at establishing laws that guarantee citizenship rights for the elderly. The following stand out in this context: the Statute of the Elderly[7] ; Active ageing: a health policy[8] ; and the National Health Policy for the Elderly[9] . However, even with the publication of these provisions, these policies still fall short in terms of the Brazilian reality, which means that there are still many situations in which the elderly are disrespected.

Providing care for the elderly is a challenging proposition given the diversity of health limitations found in this population. In addition to this, the prospect of active ageing, with the proposal of appropriate lifestyle habits and preventative measures for health problems, is inadequate. This is evidenced in a study carried out in Campinas-SP, which found a balance between active and sedentary elderly people, according to the criteria adopted in that study .[10]

In view of the above, the research questions set out in this book were established:

- What is the sociodemographic and health profile of the elderly linked to the ESF in Natal and Santa Cruz?

- What is the association between quality of life and the sociodemographic and health aspects of these elderly people?

To this end, the following statistical hypotheses were drawn up:

Null hypothesis (H^0): Quality of life is not associated with the sociodemographic and health aspects of elderly people linked to the ESF.

Alternative hypothesis (H^1): Quality of life is associated with the sociodemographic and health aspects of elderly people linked to the ESF.

Why explore Quality of Life?

The personal motivation for carrying out the research is based on the authors' previous experience of getting closer to the reality on the ground through university extension work, in which teaching and research activities were carried out over three years to promote health and prevent illnesses in the elderly linked to the ESF. University extension is an educational, cultural and scientific mechanism that provides transformative communication between the university and the social scene[11] . It also provides the student and the members involved with practical knowledge and the skills to develop their research topic in tune with the local reality.

In the political and social context, this research was justified by the scientific evidence generated in relation to the local and global context regarding care for the elderly and morbidities related to the ageing process. In this way, it raises public policy interests, in addition to the potential positive impacts of improved life expectancy in Brazil and worldwide, with a better levelling out of QoL in this age group .[12]

As far as the Brazilian context is concerned, the National Agenda of Health Research Priorities (ANPPS) highlights the importance given to diseases prevalent in the elderly, as well as their problems that are linked to the ageing process. This scenario highlights the scientific potential that the elderly population currently generates, as well as indicating huge investments in research and technologies with a view to maintaining the QoL of this public .[13]

With the increase in the elderly population and, proportionally, the dynamics of health services and establishments, there is a tendency towards fragilisation and aggravation of the difficulties already present in the national reality, caused by the high demand for elderly people in these services, as well as their prolonged time in hospital. In this sense, the evidence and relevance of this research is justified, in the sense of proposing mechanisms to mitigate the problems, reducing overcrowding in institutions .[14]

Diseases and limitations imposed or aggravated by advancing age are considered to have a great potential negative impact on QoL[15] . In view of this impact, attention is drawn to the parameters pertinent to the vulnerability of the elderly, since this is identified precisely by the burden of diseases, malnutrition, debility, as well as progressive, with advancing age[16] . This raises the question of how the elderly live with these morbidities and the impact they have on their way of life.

Therefore, combining sociodemographic and health aspects with the level of care provided by the ESF to these elderly people becomes a relevant indicator when analysing the extent to which one or more of these aspects influence the QoL of the elderly.

This research is based on the care model advocated at national level (SUS), carrying out a survey in a local universe, in environments that are peculiar to a state capital (Natal) and a municipality located in the interior of the state (Santa Cruz). This study is also justified by the fact that it will bring benefits to elderly people treated in primary care, with a possible improvement in quality of life, given its initial diagnosis and subsequent planning of interventions.

It is also justified by the need to investigate the factors that determine the QoL of the elderly and their vulnerability, in order to create a profile of the aspects that make them up. In this way, it will be possible to compare these profiles in different scenarios in order to propose future interventions aimed at improving the health aspects of this age group in the context of primary health care.

The study therefore set out to analyse the association between sociodemographic aspects and health with the quality of life of elderly people linked to the ESF. In order to achieve this objective, the following stages were established for the study:

1. To characterise the elderly in the ESF in Natal and Santa Cruz, in Rio Grande do Norte/Brazil, in terms of sociodemographic and health aspects;
2. To compare the domains and dimensions of the QoL of the elderly in the ESF in the municipalities of Natal and Santa Cruz;
3. To verify, in Natal and Santa Cruz, the association between the

domains and dimensions of QoL and sociodemographic and health aspects.

References

1. Albuquerque ER, Alves EF. Analysis of bibliographic production on the quality of life of patients with chronic wounds. Revista saúde e pesquisa. 2011; 4(2): 147-52.

2. Lucas LS, Martins JT, Robazzi MLCC. Quality of life of patients with lower limb wounds - leg ulcers. Ciência e enfermagem. 2008; 14(1): 43-52.

3. Martins, JJ. Schneider DG, Coelho FL, Nascimento ERP, Alburqueque GL, Erdmann AL, et al. Quality of life among elderly people receiving home care services. Acta paulista de enfermagem. 2014; 22(3): 265-71.

4. Vitorino LM, Paskulin LMG, Vianna LAC. Quality of life of seniors living in the community and in long term care facilities: a comparative study. Latin American Journal of Nursing. 2013; 21: 3-11.

5. Cameron, ID, Fairhall N, Langron C, Lockwood K, Monaghan N, Aggar C, et al. A multifactorial interdisciplinary intervention reduces frailty in older people: randomised trial. BMC Medicine. 2013; 11(65): 1-10.

6. Costa Neto AM, Azevedo GAV, Santos AG, Costa CPB. Habits of life and performance of elderly in basic activities of daily life. Journal of

Nursing UFPE Online. 2013; 7(7): 4663-9.

7. Brazil. Ministry of Health. Statute of the Elderly. Brasília (DF). 2003.

8. World Health Organisation (WHO). Active ageing: a health policy, Brasília (DF): PAHO; 2005.

9. Brazil. Ministry of Health. Ordinance No. 2.528, of 19 October 2006. Approves the National Health Policy for the Elderly. Brasília (DF): Ministry of Health. 2006.

10. Bez JPO, Neri AL. Gait speed, grip strength and perceived health in the elderly: data from the FIBRA Campinas network, São Paulo, Brazil. Ciência e Saúde. 2014; 19(8): 3343-53.

11. Pereira JL, Vieira VL, Jaime PC. Considerations on interdisciplinarity based on testimonies from participants in the nutrition team of the "Scientific Flag" university extension project. Demetra. 2013; 8(2): 183-95.

12. Faller JW, Melo WA, Versa GLGS, Marcon SS. Quality of life of elderly people registered with the Family Health Strategy in Foz do Iguaçu-PR. Anna Nery School. 2010; 14(4): 803-10.

13. Brazil. Ministry of Health. National agenda of health research priorities. Brasília: Ministry of Health; 2011.

14. Bajotto AP, Witter A, Mahmud SJ, Sirena S, Goldim JR. Profile of

elderly patients cared for by a home care programme of the Unified Health System in Porto Alegre, RS. Revista HCPA. 2012; 32(3): 311-17.

15. Pinto JM, Neri AL. Factors associated with low life satisfaction in community-dwelling elderly: FIBRA Study. Caderno de Saúde Pública. 2013; 29(12): 2447-58.

16. Romera L, Orfila F, Segura JM, Ramirez A, Moller M, Fabra ML, et al. Effectiveness of a primary care based multifactorial intervention to improve frailty parameters in the elderly: a randomised clinical trial: rationale and study design. BMC Geriatrics. 2014; 14(125): 1-13.

CHAPTER 3

The Methodological Path of the Study

Methodological Design

The work developed and presented in this book is an analytical, cross-sectional study with a quantitative approach, which was carried out in the communities of Igapó, in the northern part of the municipality of Natal, Rio Grande do Norte (RN), the Dner neighbourhood and the Physiotherapy School Clinic, in the municipality of Santa Cruz, RN, Brazil. The time frame of the study was December 2015 to March 2016.

Between 2013 and 2016, two projects were developed involving teaching, research and extension in these communities. Researchers were initially involved in the activities, participating in the planning and execution of the actions.

The initial project was entitled "Projeto Cuidado ao Idoso na Comunidade" (Care for the Elderly in the Community Project) and took place exclusively in primary care. It became international and extended to other levels of care in 2014, under the title "Atenção à Saúde do Idoso na Estratégia Saúde da Família no Brasil e Portugal: proposta de avaliação e intervenção multidimensional" (Care for the Elderly in the Family Health Strategy in Brazil and Portugal: a proposal for multidimensional evaluation and intervention), which is still being developed today.

The choice of municipalities was influenced by the presence of research and extension projects in them. The researchers also realised that it was appropriate to carry out the study between the two municipalities, as they have different socio-cultural and demographic characteristics, due to the fact that Natal is a large city (capital of the state) and Santa Maria is a large city (capital of the state).

Cruz, a municipality located in the interior of the state and with a smaller population.

Natal is a Brazilian municipality, characterised by being the capital of the state of Rio Grande do Norte (RN), with an estimated population of 862,044 inhabitants in 2014[1] . The Family Health Unit (USF) in the Igapó neighbourhood covers three areas and is divided into 15 micro-areas, with three teams registered with the municipality's ESF (one for each area). The fortnightly meetings with the elderly are held in a space donated by the local parish, due to the unavailability of suitable physical space in the USF itself. As professional support, the elderly in this scenario receive intervention basically from the ESF team, through their CHWs, undergraduate nursing students from UFRN, postgraduate nursing and nutrition students from UFRN, always under the coordination of one of the service's nurses.

Santa Cruz, a Brazilian municipality, is located 115 kilometres from the state capital (Natal). It is in the Potiguar mesoregion, with an estimated population of 38,538 inhabitants in 2014[1] . The USF in the Dner neighbourhood has one team that covers the area of the neighbourhood. Weekly activities with the elderly take place inside the USF itself in a space that is available. In addition to these activities, there are elderly people involved in activities at the Physiotherapy School Clinic run by the UFRN's Trairi Faculty of Science and Health (FACISA). The elderly in Santa Cruz receive interventions and multi-professional support from undergraduate students in physiotherapy, nutrition and nursing, linked to the subjects offered at that health institution. The elderly are monitored through voluntary registration at the Physiotherapy School Clinic. Stretching and warm-up activities are carried out on the floor and in the pool.

From participants to sample

Participants included elderly people linked to the ESF in the Igapó neighbourhood in the municipality of Natal, the Dner neighbourhood and users of the Physiotherapy School Clinic at the Trairi Faculty of Health Sciences (FACISA), both in Santa Cruz.

It should be noted that this study is the initial stage of a case-control type study, in which a proposal was presented to the elderly people from the two municipalities surveyed, in which they were offered a plan with various multicentre interventions aimed at improving their QoL. A group of 60 elderly people was formed, 30 of whom belonged to Igapó (Natal) and the other 30 to Santa Cruz (Dner and Clínica Escola de Fisioterapia), making up the case or intervention group.

After characterising these individuals, another group (the control group) was formed with the same n (60 elderly people), taking into account their respective municipalities, as well as five sociodemographic characteristics, in order to match the sample. The aim of this large study carried out in parallel is to verify the impact generated by interventions focussed on the demands of the elderly raised at this initial stage. Based on these, activities will be developed that seek to improve the aspects considered to be deficient, as well as maintaining the best aspects assessed.

Therefore, the total n obtained for the sample was due to the need to achieve statistical representativeness, in addition to meeting the requirements of the chosen methodology, in this case the case-control study.

It should also be noted that all the elderly, including those in the control group, received the same invitation to receive the interventions, allowing them freedom of choice. For the purposes of this study, we simply considered the total number of 120 elderly people, divided according to their research settings, with all individuals being assessed without pairing criteria.

Inclusion and exclusion criteria

In order to be included in the study, participants had to be aged 60 or over, in line with the Statute of the Elderly[2] , which considers individuals in this age group to be elderly in Brazil; be registered with the health unit in their municipality as a client at the time of collection; have cognitive ability, measured using the MMSE screening instrument, which has a cut-off point of 17 points for individuals with 3 years or less of schooling (low schooling) and 24 points for those with 4 years or more of schooling[3] . Individuals who did not meet these criteria were excluded from the study.

As a result, two elderly people from Natal and one from Santa Cruz were excluded because they did not meet the cut-off point for the MMSE. Two participants from Natal and three from Santa Cruz were approached and then excluded from the study because they were younger than the age established for this study.

Collection instruments used

The instruments selected for data collection were: the demographic data and pain characteristics questionnaire, which addresses the sociodemographic information of the elderly, such as gender, age group, marital status, as well as information regarding the presence and intensity of pain and diseases in the elderly; and the validated Brazilian version of the quality of life questionnaire Medical Outcomes Short-Form Health Survey (SF-36), made up of eight domains and two dimensions referring to QoL, with 36 questions aimed at the scalar measurement of each of them, through a scoring scale ranging from zero to one hundred (0 to 100) for each domain or dimension. The questions in the instrument refer to activities that the elderly person could or could not carry out, considering their degree of difficulty in doing so, as well as social and family activities, whether or not these are affected by physical or psychological limitations or any health problems .[4]

Indicators and variables explored

To present the results, the choice of indicators and variables was based on the content of each instrument used, as well as the aim of this study. Thus, the sociodemographic characterisation addresses the age group, considering the elderly to be aged 60 or over. The point dividing the sample between younger and older elderly people was determined by the median of the age values found. As for schooling, the elderly who reported up to three years of study were considered to have a low level, according to the parameters of the Mini Mental State Examination (MMSE). The presence or absence of activity refers to whether or not the elderly person has any kind of occupation (paid or unpaid).

When characterising health aspects, acute pain was considered to be present for less than six months and chronic pain was considered to be present for more than six months[5] . The same criterion of chronicity was applied to the variable asking about the presence of chronic diseases. The variable "other illnesses" refers to acute illnesses. The other variables were considered self-explanatory in the table or have already been described elsewhere.

Collecting information

Data collection took place on pre-determined days, targeted at the activities of the elderly groups, as well as through an active search in the study community, followed by an unannounced home visit. This search was carried out with the help of Community Health Agents (CHAs) linked to the Igapó ESF and Dner, as they had knowledge of the individuals living in the area. The collection process continued until the number of elderly people reached 120 (n= 120).

The researchers

The researchers were nurses and a nutritionist, undergraduate and postgraduate students in nursing and health sciences. Before the data was collected, the interviewers underwent a training process on the selected instruments. To this end, they studied the instruments in advance, using material provided, and then discussed them in detail. A "pre-test" was then carried out by simulating the application of the forms among the researchers.

After the simulation, the training was finalised with feedback, rediscussing the elements of the forms. This way, only those individuals who had undergone this process took part.

Statistical analysis and presentation of the data collected

Microsoft Excel 2013 and Statistical Package for the Social Sciences (SPSS) 20.0 were used to tabulate and analyse the data. For the nominal and ordinal variables relating to sociodemographic and health characterisation, the Pearson Chi-squared non-parametric test was applied to check the significance of the dispersion between the compared variables. For variables with frequencies of less than five ($n<5$), Fisher's Exact Test was used, which is a more appropriate test for this situation.

The sample was tested for normality and found not to be normal. Therefore, the Mann-Whitney U-test was used to test the scalar variables in this study in relation to the SF-36 scale. This is the test of choice for this analysis because it is non-parametric and considers the analysis between independent variables, i.e. the SF-36 domains and the study sites. The Kruskal Wallis test was used to compare the means of variables with more than two categories. A 95% Confidence Interval (CI) was adopted and findings with a p-value < 0.05 were significant.

To answer the research objectives, the two statistical hypotheses were tested: H^0 : considering that sociodemographic and health aspects are not associated with the quality of life of the elderly linked to the FHS (p-value > 0.05). Alternative hypothesis H1: sociodemographic and health aspects are associated with the quality of life of elderly people linked to the FHS (p-value < 0.05).

The data was presented in tables when it involved analyses of categorical variables and tables for the presentation of scalar measures. When frequency values were presented, the results were represented by the letter "n" (total number found).

Ethical and legal aspects of research

In accordance with Resolution 466/12 of the National Health Council, which deals with studies with human beings[6] , this research was approved by the Research Ethics Committee of the Onofre Lopes University Hospital (CEP/HUOL) under Certificate of Submission for Ethical Appraisal (CAAE) number 21996313.7.0000.5537. Before the interviews were carried out, the participants were presented with the Informed Consent Form (ICF), which they then signed. The Primary Care service of the Igapó ESF granted the researchers prior authorisation to carry out the study in their area.

References

1. Brazilian Institute of Geography and Statistics (IBGE). Demographic Census 2014. Population estimates for Brazilian municipalities. Rio de Janeiro: Brazilian Institute of Geography and Statistics; 2014.

2. Brazil. Ministry of Health. Statute of the Elderly. Brasília (DF); 2013.

3. Murden, RA, McRae TD, Kaner S, Bucknam ME. Mini-Mental State Exam Scores Vary with Education in Blacks and Whites. Journal American

Geriatrics. 1991; 39: 149-55.

4. Ciconelli, RM. Ferraz MB, Santos W, Meinão I, Quaresma MR. Translation into Portuguese and validation of the SF-36 generic quality of life questionnaire (Brazil SF-36). Brazilian Journal of Rheumatology. 1999; 39(3): 143-50.

5. NANDA International, Inc. NANDA International Nursing Diagnoses 2012-2014, Translated by: Regina Machado Garcez. Editora Artmed; 2013.

6. Brazil. Federal Official Gazette. Resolution 466, of 12 December 2012. Federal Official Gazette: Ministry of Health; 2012.

CHAPTER 4

Results and discussion regarding the QoL of the elderly in the ESF

A total of 120 elderly people registered with the ESFs took part in the study, with a predominance of females, young elderly people who, although retired, still had daily activities. This profile was similar when analysing the two scenarios in isolation. In terms of years of schooling, the total sample showed a slight majority with low levels of schooling. The same was true of marital status, since just over half had a partner. When looking at family income, there was a significant difference between the cities (p <0.001), with the majority in Natal earning up to one minimum wage, while the majority in Santa Cruz earned more than one minimum wage.

Table 1 - Sociodemographic characterisation of the elderly, according to place of study. Natal and Santa Cruz, Rio Grande do Norte, Brazil, 2016 (n=120)

Sociodemographic characterisation		Christmas		Santa Cruz		Total		Chi-Square
		n	%	n	%	n	%	ρ-value
Sex	Female	50	41,7	50	41,7	100	83,3	1,000
	Male	10	8,3	10	8,3	20	16,7	
Age group	60 to 75 years old	44	36,7	50	41,7	94	78,3	0,184
	76 to 91 years old	16	13,3	10	8,3	26	21,7	
Education	Up to 3 years	31	25,8	30	25,0	61	50,8	0,855
	> 3 years	29	24,2	30	25,0	59	49,2	
Marital	With company	29	24,2	34	28,3	63	52,	0,361

status							5	
	Without company	31	25,8	26	21,7	57	47,5	
Family income	Up to 1 minimum wage	36	30,0	16	13,3	52	43,3	**< 0,001**
	> 1 minimum wage	24	20,0	44	36,7	68	56,7	
Who do you live with	With a partner	23	19,2	31	25,8	54	45,0	
	Children/grandchildren	25	20,8	21	17,5	46	38,3	0,060
	Alone	12	10,0	5	4,2	17	14,2	
	Others*	0	0,0	3	2,5	3	2,5	
Work situation	Retired	51	42,5	43	35,8	94	78,3	
	Look after the house	8	6,7	13	10,8	21	17,5	0,276
	Away	0	0,0	1	0,8	1	0,8	
Has activity	Yes	58	48,3	57	47,5	115	95,8	1,000
	No	2	1,7	3	2,5	5	4,2	

Source: own research. Note: * Brother/cousin/friend

Analysing the health aspects (Table 2), considering the total sample, we found the presence of pain, mainly chronic and of moderate intensity. When analysing the reported sites of pain, the dorsal region stood out, followed by the lower limbs and upper limbs. With regard to the presence of chronic diseases, 88.3% of the elderly said they had them, while 60% said they had no other types of non-chronic diseases. In view of this, attention was drawn to the use of medication, which was present in 85% of the elderly. Despite the differences, none of the variables showed any significant difference.

Table 2 - Characterisation of the health aspects of the elderly,

according to place of study. Natal and Santa Cruz, Rio Grande do Norte, Brazil, 2016 (n=120)

Characterisation of health aspects		Place of study Christmas		Santa Cruz		Total		Chi-squared p-value
		n	%	n	%	n	%	
Pain in the last week	Yes	45	37,5	43	35,8	88	73,3	0,680
	No	15	12,5	17	14,2	32	26,7	
Type of pain	Chronicle	33	27,5	31	25,8	64	53,3	0,822
	Acute	13	10,8	12	10,0	25	20,8	
	Absent	14	11,7	17	14,2	31	25,8	
Pain intensity	Lightweight	8	6,7	10	8,3	18	15,0	0,825
	Moderate	21	17,5	19	15,8	40	33,3	
	Intense	17	14,2	14	11,7	31	25,8	
Place of pain	Back	12	10,0	17	14,2	29	24,2	0,502
	MMII	14	11,7	10	8,3	24	20,0	
	MMSS	4	3,3	6	5,0	10	8,3	
	Generalised	4	3,3	5	4,2	9	7,5	
	Lumbar	6	5,0	2	1,7	8	6,7	
	Painless	14	11,7	17	14,2	31	25,8	
Chronic diseases	Yes	56	46,7	50	41,7	106	88,3	0,153*
	No	4	3,3	10	8,3	14	11,7	
Other diseases	Yes	27	22,5	21	17,5	48	40,0	0,295
	No	33	27,5	39	32,5	72	60,0	
Uses medication	Yes	55	45,8	47	39,2	102	85,0	0,410
	No	5	4,2	13	10,8	18	15,0	

Source: Own research. Note: * Fisher's Exact Test.

Table 1 shows the QoL scores of the elderly. When analysing the SF-36 domains, it was noted that the mean values were similar when comparing the two municipalities. With regard to the best domains, the emotional aspect stood out, with an average of 78.3 (+39.2) in Natal and 76.6 (+40.8) in Santa Cruz, followed by the functional aspect, with an average of 63.1 (+26.4) in Natal and 64.3 (+26.2) in Santa Cruz. There was no significant difference between the two cities.

The worst averages were for pain, 36.3 (+21.8) in Natal and 33.2 (+20.6) in Santa Cruz, followed by general state of health, 44.6 (+16.3) in Natal and 39.5 (+16.3) in Santa Cruz.

It can be seen that in certain domains Natal had a higher average: emotional aspects, average 78.3 (+ 39.2); vitality, average 56.9 (+ 15.4); general state of health, average 44.6 (+ 16.3); and bodily pain, average 36.3 (+ 21.8). In the other domains, Santa Cruz was the scenario that stood out: functional mean 64.3, (+ 26.2); mental health, mean 59.6 (+ 8.1); physical, mean 59.1 (+ 45.8); and social function, mean 49.6 (+ 13.0).

With regard to the mental and physical health dimensions, there was a similar balance, with no significance when comparing the two scenarios, with ρ-values of 0.457 and 0.665, respectively. The average of the total sample for the two dimensions was: mental health, with an average of 56.7 (+ 10.1) and physical health, with an average of 50.6 (+ 10.6).

Chart 1 - Analysis of the quality of life of the elderly, according to place of study. Natal and Santa Cruz, Rio Grande do Norte, Brazil, 2016 (n=120)

Quality of Life (SF-36)		Natal Mean (SD)	Santa Cruz Mean (SD)	Mann-Whitney U (ρ-value)	Total Mean (SD)
Dom	Emotional aspect	78,3 (39,2)	76,6 (40,8)	0,924	77,5 (39,9)
	Functional	63,1 (26,4)	64,3	0,809	63,7

ai			(26,2)		(26,2)
ns	**Mental health**	58,0(11,6)	59,6 (8,0)	0,844	58,8 (10,0)
	Physical	54,6 (47,2)	59,1 (45,8)	0,622	56,9 (46,4)
	Vitality	56,9(15,4)	54,6 (14,9)	0,376	55,9(15,2)
	General state of health	44,6(16,3)	39,5 (16,3)	0,083	42,1 (16,4)
	Social function	48,9(16,1)	49,6 (13,0)	0,372	49,2 (14,6)
	Pain	36,3 (21,8)	33,2 (20,6)	0,406	34,7 (21,2)
Dimensions	**Mental health**	57,3 (9,6)	56,0 (10,6)	0,457	56,7 (10,1)
	Physics	51,1 (10,4)	50,1 (10,9)	0,665	50,6 (10,6)
Total score		55,1 (8,8)	54,6 (10,2)	0,902	54,9 (9,5)

Source: own research.

The association between sociodemographic aspects and the QoL of the elderly is described in Table 3. Only the domains and dimensions that were significant in at least one city are shown.

In Santa Cruz, there was an association between age group and the functional (**ρ-value** 0.03), emotional (**ρ-value** 0.04) and physical (**ρ-value** 0.04) domains, with younger elderly people showing better averages. Also in Santa Cruz, there was an association between marital status and the functional (**ρ-value** 0.037) and emotional (**ρ-value** 0.043) domains, showing better averages in those with a partner, and between income and the functional domain (ρ-value 0.008) in favour of higher income.

As for Natal, the significant association appeared in the age group only with the emotional domain (ρ-value 0.04), showing a better score in older people. The variable has activity was also significantly associated with this city in the functional aspect (p-value 0.034), for those who had activity.

Table 3 - Association between sociodemographic aspects and QOL in the elderly. Natal and Santa Cruz, Rio Grande do Norte, Brazil, 2016 (n=120)

Socio-demographic aspects	Quality of Life							
	Domains				Dimensions			
	Functional		Emotional		Physical Health		Total score	
Age group	**Christmas**	**S. Cruz**	**Christmas**	**S. Cruz**	**Christmas**	**S. Cruz**	**Christmas**	**S. Cross**
60 to 75 years old	65,4	67,2	72,0	82,0	51,7	51,4	54,7	56,1
76 to 91 years old	56,9	50,0	95,8	50,0	49,5	43,7	56,1	47,1
ρ-value**	0,287	**0,032**	**0,028**	**0,040**	0,461	**0,042**	0,569	**0,014**
Marital status								
With company	65,0	69,7	80,5	87,2	49,6	51,3	54,1	56,6
Without company	61,4	57,3	76,3	62,8	52,5	48,8	56,0	52,0
p-value**	0,568	**0,037**	0,681	**0,043**	0,286	0,374	0,317	0,107
Family income								
Up to 1 salary	60,5	50,6	75,9	60,4	50,3	47,2	54,6	50,4
> 1 Salary	67,1	69,3	81,9	82,6	52,4	51,2	55,7	56,2
ρ-value**	0,368	**0,008**	0,697	0,060	0,441	0,216	0,629	0,056
Has activity								
Yes	64,5	64,6	77,6	77,1	51,3	49,7	55,3	54,2
No	22,5	58,3	66,6	-	44,5	58,6	48,0	59,0
ρ-value**	**0,03**	0,65	0,547	0,798	0,36	0,209	0,307	0,377

4	3		6

Source: own research. Note: **Mann-Whitney U-test.

The association between health aspects and QoL (Table 4) shows a significant association in Santa Cruz between the aspect "pain in the last week" and the functional (ρ-value 0.013), bodily pain (ρ-value <0.001), emotional (ρ-value 0.019) and mental health (ρ-value 0.026) domains.

Also in the municipality of Santa Cruz, there was a significant association between the type of pain and the functional (ρ-value 0.044) and emotional (ρ-value <0.001) domains, and between the variable use of medication and the functional domain (ρ-value 0.020).

In Natal, the only significant association was between the type of pain and the functional domain (ρ-value 0.040).

Table 4 - Association between aspects of health and QoL in the elderly. Natal and Santa Cruz, Rio Grande do Norte, Brazil, 2016 (n=120)

Health aspects	**Quality of Life**						**Dimension**	
	Domains							
	Functional		**Body Pain**		**Emotional**		**Mental Health**	
Pain in the last week	**Christmas**	**S Cruz**	**Christmas**	**S. Cruz**	**Christmas**	**S. Cruz**	**Christmas**	**S. Cruz**
Yes	61,2	59,4	39,1	42,8	74,1	69,0	56,3	54,3
No	69,0	76,7	28,0	8,8	91,1	96,1	60,5	60,2
ρ-value**	0,342	**0,013**	0,115	**<0,001**	0,161	**0,019**	0,124	**0,026**
Type of pain								
Chronicle	55,4	60,3	42,1	41,3	64,6	69,9	54,6	53,8
Acute	71,9	57,1	34,6	46,7	-	66,6	59,8	55,7
Absent	73,2	76,7	24,3	8,8	90,5	96,1	61,4	60,2
ρ-value***	**0,040**	**0,044**	0,054	**<0,001**	0,007	0,062	0,052	0,080

Use medicines								
Yes	62,1	60,2	36,7	33,4	78,2	73,7	57,2	55,6
No	75,0	79,2	32,0	32,3	80,0	97,2	58,4	57,4
ρ-value**	0,403	**0,020**	0,603	0,978	0,856	0,275	0,795	0,794

Source: own research. Note: **Mann-Whitney U-test; ***Kruskal Wallis test.

Figure 1 shows the association between QoL domains and sociodemographic and health variables in the municipalities.

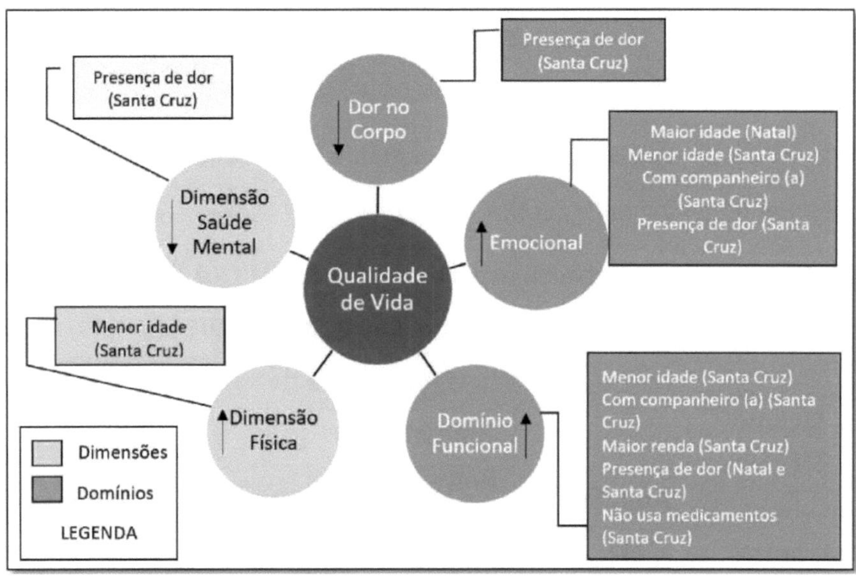

Figure 1 - Association between aspects of health and QoL in the elderly. Natal and Santa Cruz, Rio Grande do Norte, Brazil, 2016 (n=60)

Source: Own research

Table 5 shows the association between sociodemographic aspects and QoL, considering the sample as a single population and not divided by city. There was an association between age group and family income and the functional domain, in favour of the younger elderly (mean 67.3 and **ρ-value**

= 0.022) and those with a higher income (mean 68.5 and **ρ-value** = 0.018). Family income was also associated with body pain, but in favour of older people with lower incomes (mean 39 and **ρ-value**= 0.029). The other domains had no significant association.

Table 5 - Association between sociodemographic aspects and QOL in the elderly, according to the total sample. Natal and Santa Cruz, Rio Grande do Norte, Brazil, 2016 (n=120)

Sociodemographic aspects	**Quality of Life Domains**	
	Functional	**Body Pain**
Age group		
60 to 75 years old	67,3	35,2
76 to 91 years old	57,9	33,9
ρ-value*	**0,022**	0,849
Family income		
Up to 1 salary	57,5	39
> Salary	68,5	31,4
ρ-value*	**0,018**	**0,029**

Source: own research. Note: *Mann-Whitney U-test.

The association between aspects of health and QoL in the elderly, considering the sample as just one population, showed a significant association between the variable "pain in the last week" and the functional (**ρ-value** 0.016), bodily pain (<0.001), emotional (**ρ-value** 0.007) and mental health (**ρ-value** 0.008) domains, with only the bodily pain domain showing a better average for those who had pain in the last week. With regard to the type of pain, there was also an association with the functional (ρ-value 0.008), bodily pain (ρ-value <0.001), emotional (ρ-value 0.004) and mental health (ρ-value 0.007) domains, with better averages for acute pain compared to chronic pain, except for the bodily pain domain.

With regard to chronic illnesses and the use of medication, significance was only found in the functional domain (ρ-value 0.027 and ρ-value 0.015, respectively), with better averages for those who did not have chronic illnesses and who did not use medication.

Table 6 - Association between aspects of health and QoL in the elderly, according to the total sample. Natal and Santa Cruz, Rio Grande do Norte, Brazil, 2016 (n=120).

Health aspects	Quality of Life			
	Domains			Dimension
	Functional	**Body Pain**	**Emotional**	**Mental Health**
Pain in the last week				
Yes	60,3	40,9	71,6	55,3
No	73,1	17,8	93,7	60,3
ρ-value*	**0,016**	**<0,001**	**0,007**	**0,008**
Type of pain				
Chronicle	57,8	41,7	67,2	54,2
Acute	64,8	40,4	84	57,8
Absent	75,1	15,8	93,5	60,7
ρ-value**	**0,008**	**<0,001**	**0,004**	**0,007**
Chronic diseases				
Yes	61,8	35	78	57
No	78,2	32,8	73,8	53,9
ρ-value*	**0,027**	0,753	0,829	0,615
Use medicines				
Yes	61,2	35,2	76,1	56,5
No	78,0	32,2	85,2	57,7
ρ-value*	**0,015**	0,021	0,305	0,834

Source: own research. Note: *Mann-Whitney U-test; **Kruskal Wallis test.

The scientific context of the findings of this research

The purpose of this study was to analyse sociodemographic and health aspects and to compare QoL associated with these aspects among the elderly in the municipalities of Natal and Santa Cruz. The predominance of women in the sample is in line with the results found in the literature[1,2,3] . Although a majority in both municipalities, gender was not significantly associated with QoL.

In contrast to this study, a similar profile carried out in Brazil showed better QoL scores in men than in women, although they had a greater burden of illness, physical limitations and depressive symptoms[4] . In Natal and Santa Cruz, there was a predominance of chronic diseases in women.

In relation to Natal and Santa Cruz in terms of chronic diseases and conditions, there was a balance between the cities, with Santa Cruz having a slightly lower number of elderly sufferers. A cohort study carried out in Spain showed that these comorbidities have a major impact on the QoL of the elderly, particularly disability and physical dependence[5] . In contrast to this finding, Natal and Santa Cruz alone showed no significant association between the presence of chronic diseases and QoL. However, considering the total sample, i.e. the combination of the two scenarios, there was a significant association between the functional domain and the absence of chronic diseases.

Results found[6-8] show that the impact of diseases and comorbidities can be reduced by changing lifestyle habits towards healthier behaviours, such as improving nutrition and starting physical activity. In addition, active elderly people generally have a lower disease burden and improved health compared to those who are idle[9] . This highlights the importance of interventions to encourage exercise and healthy eating.

In this follow-up, it was noted that Natal and Santa Cruz obtained the functional domain among the best evaluated through the SF-36. Functionality was associated with QoL in a study of elderly Canadians, and the association was significant[10] . Another study of institutionalised elderly people found that functional behaviour ranged from average to good, with the decline in this aspect being linked to advancing age[3] . This result is in line with what was found in Santa Cruz and in the total sample, in which there was a strong association between the functional domain and age group, with the best average being found in young elderly people. When the physical dimension was assessed, the behaviour was similar to that of functionality.

In this sense, a study[11] found that interventions aimed at promoting physical activity in the elderly, even if the activity is infrequent, are effective. Another study[12] found that motivation was responsible for positive results in terms of preventing disabilities and other problems, since it promotes the autonomy of the elderly in their social and functional context.

Still thinking about QoL, mental health stood out in both cities, with results above the scale's median. The relationship between mental health with depression makes this disease a focus in the literature, given the need to evaluate mental and emotional aspects, relating them to the QoL of the elderly[4] . Recent literature has found data indicating a worsening of QoL in Iranian elderly people with depressive symptoms, when compared to elderly people without symptoms[1] . In Santa Cruz, the domain of emotional aspects was strongly associated in favour of the younger age group, with the presence of company and the absence of pain. In Natal, there was a strong association between the same domain in favour of the older elderly and in the total sample, in favour of the absence of pain.

A study carried out in 2015[13] , which evaluated elderly people, showed higher scores in the mental and physical health domains, similar to the data in this study. An international cohort study found a relationship between improved health-related QoL and reduced depression[14] . It should be emphasised that in Santa Cruz, emotional aspects were negatively and significantly associated with older people and the absence of a partner.

As a result, it was realised that family support has an influence on QoL and has a direct and positive effect on the emotional aspect[15] . This is in line with a Polish study which, after investigating family emotional support, found a significant negative difference between institutionalised and non-institutionalised elderly people[16] . In this study, just over half of the sample had a partner, and a balance was observed between the cities. It was also found that most of the elderly lived with family members, including children and grandchildren, which could be a positive factor for QoL.

Another important factor that alters the QoL of the elderly, in addition to family support, is social interaction within their daily lives[17] . The World

Health Organisation (WHO) defines active ageing in a comprehensive way, which includes health opportunities, the political and social context, and having the right to exercise their citizenship in a participatory way .[18]

In the United States of America (USA), a population-based study revealed a proportional inverse relationship between social support in the elderly and the level of vulnerability that has a significant impact on QoL[19] . In China, it was also found that the score in the social domain decreased when the vulnerability of the elderly increased[20] . In this study, the social domain was one of the lowest averages among the domains in both cities, but there was no significance with sociodemographic and health characteristics.

It is therefore important to promote social interaction between the elderly and society, regardless of age, gender and culture. Studies carried out in Brazil have linked the presence of illnesses and comorbidities to social isolation, since the elderly do not leave the house. By not leaving the house, the elderly are potentially at risk of reduced socialisation, with a negative influence on their QoL[17] . This identifies the relationship between the social and physical domains.

In view of the above, there is a need to plan and implement measures to increase QoL and provide active ageing for the elderly. To this end, the importance and increasingly frequent use of technologies as tools for interventions in the elderly has been noted, as studies have shown results that improve cognition, social inclusion, disease prevention and health maintenance[21-23] Strategies to promote coping, improve self-esteem and adapt to activities of daily living are presented to provide healthy ageing .[13]

In this study, it was clear that the elderly in both municipalities, although retired, were active in some way. Despite this, the scores for the physical and functional domains were classified as average and good respectively. Thus, there is a clear need for a detailed investigation into the type of activity carried out by the elderly, added to the complexity, so that it is possible to assess the suitability of their movements and measure their health benefits, in order to improve QoL scores.

This study suggests the planning of new interventions to improve the social domain and maintain the other domains. As already discussed, the use of technological resources and the digital inclusion of the elderly has emerged as the methodology of choice for working on interventions in this direction.

As for limitations, the following stand out: the cross-sectional design, the long collection period. The difficulty of the study was mainly due to the unhealthy conditions faced by the researchers in the active search for participants.

CHAPTER 5

Conclusion and final considerations

This research revealed that the characteristics inherent to Natal and Santa Cruz were not significantly associated with the QoL observed when comparing the two scenarios. However, it was important to profile the main aspects in order to deepen the evaluation, so as to positively interfere in their QoL, as well as in the search to reduce their vulnerability.

It was possible to see that the emotional and functional domains showed better results, which suggests that these aspects can be taken as a basis for exploring how to promote autonomy among the elderly. It was also noted that the pain, general health and social domains had lower averages in both municipalities. This emphasises the importance of planning interventions to strengthen these sequences, as well as to maintain or improve the other domains.

With regard to the association between sociodemographic and health aspects and the QoL of the elderly, there was significance between various variables and domains. We therefore accept the alternative hypothesis (H^1), in which we consider the presence of an association between QoL and the sociodemographic and health aspects of the elderly linked to the ESF.

Given the complexity of the concept of QoL, as well as the very domains that make it up, according to the theoretical framework adopted, there is a need for greater depth and evaluation of each of these. Such research would aim to improve the accuracy of their assessment, providing precise and impactful interventions with optimum effectiveness.

References

1. Keshavarzi S, Ahmadi SM, Lankarani KB. The Impact of Depression and Malnutrition on Health-Related Quality of Life Among the Elderly Iranians. Global Journal of Health Science. 2015; 7(3): 161-70.

2. Cybulski M, Krajewska-Kulak E, Jamiolkowski J. Preferred health behaviours and quality of life of the elderly people in Poland. Clinical Interventions in Aging. 2015; 10: 1555-64.

3. Muszalik M. Kornatowski T, Zielinska H, Kediziora-Kornatowska K, Dijkstra A. Functional assessment of geriatric patients in regard to health-related quality of life (HRQoL). Clinical Interventions in Aging. 2015;10: 61-67.

4. Campos AC, Ferreira e Ferreira E, Vargas AM, Albala C. Aging, gender and quality of life (AGEQOL) study: factors associated with good quality of life in older Brazilian community dwelling adults. Health and Quality of Life Outcomes. 2014; 12(166): 1-11.

5. Forjaz MJ, Blazquez CR, Ayala A, Rodriquez VR, Cuesta JP, Gutierrez SC, et al. Chronic conditions, disability, and quality of life in older adults with multimorbidity in Spain. European Journal of Internal Medicine. 2015; 26: 17681.

6. Garin, N. Olaya B, Moneta MC, Miret M, Lobo A, Ayuso-Mateos JL, et

al. Impact of Multimorbidity on Disability and Quality of Life in the Spanish Older Population. Plos one. 2014; 9(11): 1-12.

7. Atlas A, Grimmer K, Kennedy K. Early indications that low mental quality of life scores in recently unwell older people predict downstream functional decline. Clinical Interventions in Aging. 2015; 10: 703-12.

8. Yamada Y, Merz L, Kisvetrova H. Quality of life and comorbidity among older home care clients: role of positive attitudes toward aging. Quality of Life Research. 2015; 24: 1661-67.

9. Lai CKY, Chan EA, Chin KCW. Who are the healthy active seniors? A cluster analysis. BMC Geriatrics. 2014; 14(127): 1-7.

10. Davis JC, Bryan S, Li LC, Best JR, Hsu CL, Gomez C, et al. Mobility and cognition are associated with wellbeing and health-related quality of life among older adults: a cross-sectional analysis of the Vancouver Falls Prevention Cohort. BMC Geriatrics. 2015; 15(75): 1-7.

11. Quehenberger V, Cichocki M, Krajic K. Sustainable effects of a low-threshold physical activity intervention on health-related quality of life in residential aged care. Clinical Interventions in Aging. 2014; 9: 1853-64.

12. Morgan GS, Haase AM, Campbell R, Ben-Shlomo. Physical Activity facilitation for Elders (PACE): study protocol for a randomised controlled trial. Trials. 2015; 16(91): 1-7.

13. Ziólkowski A, Blachnio A, Pachalska M. An evaluation of life satisfaction and health - Quality of life of senior citizens. Annals of Agricultural and Environmental Medicine. 2015; 22(1): 147-51.

14. Hajek, A. Brettschneider C, Ernst A, Lang C, Wiese B, Prokein J, et al. Complex coevolution of depression and health-related quality of life in old age. Quality of Life Research. 2015; 24: 2713-22.

15. Marques EMBG, Sánches CS, Vicario BP. Support as a factor promoting the quality of life of the elderly. Social Pedagogy. 2014; 23: 253-71.

16. Cybulski M, Krajewska-Kulak E, Jamiolkowski J. Preferred health behaviours and quality of life of the elderly people in Poland. Clinical Interventions in Aging. 2015; 10: 1555-64.

17. Morsch P, Pereira GN, Navarro JHN, Trevisan MD Lopes DGC, Bós AJG. Clinical and social determinants for the elderly to leave home. Caderno de Saúde Pública. 2015; 31(5): 1025-34.

18. World Health Organisation (WHO). Active aging: a policy framework. World Hearth Organisation; 2002.

19. Peek MK, Howrey BT, Ternent RS, Ray LA, Ottenbacher KJ. Social support, stressors, and frailty among older Mexican American adults. The Journals of Gerontology. 2012; 67(6): 755-64.

20. Chang YW. Chen WL, Fang WH, Yen MY, Hsieh CC, Kao TW. Frailty and Its Impact on Health Related Quality of Life: A Cross Sectional Study on Elderly Community-Dwelling Preventive Health Service Users. PLOS One. 2012; 7(5): 1-5.

21. Gustafson DH, McTavish F, Gustafson Jr DH, Mahoney JE, Johnson RA, Lee JD, et al. The effect of an information and communication technology (ICT) on older adults' quality of life: study protocol for a randomised control trial. Trials. 2015; 16(191): 1-12.

22. Callari TC, Ciairano S, Re A. Elderly-technology interaction: accessibility and acceptability of technological devices promoting motor and cognitive training. Work. 2012; 41: 362-9.

23. Hein MA, Aragaki SS. Health and ageing: a study of Brazilian master's dissertations (2000-2009). Ciência & Saúde Coletiva. 2012; 17(8): 2141-50.

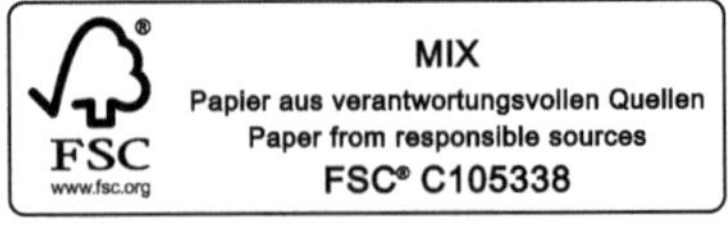

Printed by Books on Demand GmbH, Norderstedt / Germany